MASTERING THE INSULIN RESISTANCE DIET

A Comprehensive Guide to Reversing Insulin Resistance, Weight Loss, and Optimal Health

Adams .U. Morris

TABLE OF CONTENTS

CHAPTER 1

Insulin Resistance diet

In our fast-paced modern world, health concerns are prevalent, and one term that has gained significant attention is "insulin resistance." But what exactly is it, and why does it matter? Let's embark on a journey to understand this concept in simple, human terms.

The Body's Marvelous Machine:

First, we need to appreciate the incredible machine that is the human body. Imagine your body as a finely-tuned engine, running on the fuel we call food. Now, this engine relies on a substance known as insulin to make sure everything runs smoothly.

Meet Insulin:

Insulin is like the gatekeeper of your body's cells. When you eat, your body breaks down the food into sugars, mainly glucose. Glucose is the primary source of energy for your cells. However, glucose can't just enter your cells on its own. That's where insulin comes in.

Think of insulin as a key. When you eat, especially when you consume carbohydrates, your blood sugar (glucose) levels rise. This is entirely normal. However, for those with insulin resistance, the key, or insulin, doesn't work as effectively as it should.

The Lock and Key Analogy:

Let's use an analogy to illustrate this. Imagine your cells have doors, and insulin is the key that's supposed to unlock these doors, allowing glucose to enter. In a healthy system, the key (insulin) fits perfectly into the lock, and the door swings open without a hitch.

But in insulin resistance, something changes. The locks (receptors on your cells) become rusty or covered in gunk, making it hard for the key (insulin) to turn and unlock the door. As a result, your body needs to produce more and more insulin to force those doors open. This is like trying to turn a stiff key in a rusty lock – it takes a lot of effort.

A Vicious Cycle:

Now, here's where things get complicated and problematic. When your body keeps pumping out more insulin to deal with high blood sugar, it can lead to a vicious cycle. Higher insulin levels encourage your body to store more fat, especially around your abdomen. This weight gain can make insulin resistance worse, which, in turn, prompts your body to produce even more insulin.

Why Does It Matter?

At this point, you might be wondering, "So what if my cells don't let glucose in easily? Does it really matter?" The answer is a resounding yes, and here's why:

1. **Blood Sugar Rollercoaster:** Insulin resistance leads to chronically elevated blood sugar levels. Picture a rollercoaster with steep climbs and sudden drops. That's what happens to your blood sugar. These fluctuations can leave you feeling tired, irritable, and hungry shortly after eating.

2. **Weight Gain:** As mentioned earlier, insulin resistance often leads to

weight gain, particularly around your midsection. This isn't just about appearance; excess belly fat is linked to a higher risk of various health problems, including heart disease and type 2 diabetes.

3. **Type 2 Diabetes:** If insulin resistance persists, it can progress to type 2 diabetes. In diabetes, your body can't produce enough insulin to keep blood sugar in check. This can result in serious health complications like kidney disease, nerve

damage, and vision problems.

4. **Heart Health:** Insulin resistance is closely tied to heart disease. High insulin levels can lead to high blood pressure and unhealthy cholesterol levels, increasing the risk of heart attacks and strokes.

5. **Other Health Complications:** Insulin resistance has also been linked to polycystic ovary syndrome (PCOS), sleep apnea, and even certain types of cancer.

Causes and Risk Factors:

Insulin resistance isn't a one-size-fits-all condition. It can develop for various reasons, and certain factors increase your risk. Here are some common causes and risk factors:

1. **Genetics:** Some people are genetically predisposed to insulin resistance. If your family has a history of diabetes or related conditions, your risk may be higher.

2. **Lifestyle:** An unhealthy lifestyle plays a significant role. A diet high in sugary

and processed foods, combined with a lack of physical activity, can contribute to insulin resistance.

3. **Obesity:** Carrying excess weight, especially around your abdomen, is a major risk factor. Fat cells, especially in the abdominal area, release substances that can interfere with insulin's action.

4. **Inactivity:** Physical activity helps your cells become more responsive to insulin. A sedentary lifestyle, on the

other hand, can promote insulin resistance.

5. **Age:** As we age, our cells may become less responsive to insulin. This is why type 2 diabetes is more common in older adults.

6. **Hormonal Changes:** Conditions like PCOS and hormonal imbalances can contribute to insulin resistance in women.

7. **Medications:** Certain medications, such as some antipsychotic drugs and corticosteroids, can induce insulin resistance as a side effect.

Understanding these causes and risk factors is crucial because it means there are steps you can take to reduce your risk and manage insulin resistance.

Conclusion:

In essence, insulin resistance is a condition where your body's cells don't respond as effectively to insulin as they should. This can lead to a range of health problems, including high blood sugar, weight gain, and an increased risk of type 2 diabetes and heart disease.

In the following chapters, we will explore how to identify insulin resistance, what an insulin-friendly diet looks like, and lifestyle strategies to improve insulin sensitivity. Armed with this knowledge, you can take steps to take control of your health and manage insulin resistance effectively. Remember, your body is an amazing machine, and with the right care and attention, you can keep it running smoothly for years to come.

CHAPTER 2

The Role of Insulin in the Body

In Chapter 1, we dove into the concept of insulin resistance, where the body's cells don't respond effectively to insulin, a vital hormone. Now, let's explore the fundamental role that insulin plays in our bodies. Think of this chapter as an introduction to the star of the show – insulin!

The Insulin Story Begins:

To understand the significance of insulin, we need to go back to the basics of what happens when you eat. When you enjoy a meal, your digestive system gets to work, breaking down the food into its basic components. One of these components is glucose, a type of sugar that serves as the primary source of energy for your cells.

The Glucose Dilemma:

Now, here's the dilemma: Glucose is like the fuel for your body, but it can't simply enter your cells by itself. It needs an escort, and that escort is insulin.

Insulin as the Gatekeeper:

Think of insulin as a gatekeeper or a key. Your cells have doors, and insulin is the key that unlocks these doors, allowing glucose to enter. This process is essential because glucose is the energy currency your cells use to perform their various functions.

The Role of Pancreas:

So, where does insulin come from? It's produced by an amazing little organ called the pancreas. The pancreas constantly monitors the amount of glucose in your bloodstream. When you eat and your blood sugar levels rise, the pancreas gets the signal to release insulin into your bloodstream.

The Perfect Balance:

The magic lies in how insulin helps maintain balance. When you eat, especially if your meal includes carbohydrates, your blood sugar levels spike. This is a natural and necessary part of the process. However, without insulin, your blood sugar would keep rising and become dangerously high.

Insulin's Key Functions:

Now, let's break down insulin's key functions:

1. **Glucose Transport:** As mentioned, insulin acts as the key that unlocks your cells' doors. When insulin is present, your cells open up, allowing glucose to enter and be used for energy.

2. **Storage:** Insulin also has another role – it helps your body store excess glucose as glycogen in the liver and muscles. This glycogen serves as a reserve energy source for when you need it, like during exercise or between meals.

3. **Inhibits Glucose Production:** Insulin puts a

brake on your liver's glucose production. When you don't need more glucose, insulin tells your liver to stop making it.

Balancing Act:

Maintaining balanced blood sugar levels is crucial for your well-being. If your blood sugar gets too high, it can damage various organs and tissues over time. Conversely, if it drops too low, you might experience symptoms like shakiness, dizziness, and confusion.

A Dance of Hormones:

Insulin is just one player in a complex hormonal orchestra that regulates blood sugar. There are other hormones, like glucagon, that have the opposite effect of insulin. Glucagon signals your liver to release stored glucose when your blood sugar levels drop, like during fasting or intense physical activity.

Insulin Resistance and the Broken Key:

Now, remember the analogy of insulin resistance from Chapter 1? Insulin resistance occurs when the keys (insulin) don't work as effectively as they should. Imagine trying to unlock a door with a bent or rusty key – it takes more effort and doesn't always work.

In the case of insulin resistance, your body needs to produce more and more insulin to get the job done. This leads to chronically elevated insulin levels, which can have various negative consequences.

The Impact of Insulin Dysfunction:

When insulin isn't working properly, several things can happen:

1. **High Blood Sugar:** Despite the extra insulin, your blood sugar might remain high, leading to the rollercoaster effect we discussed in Chapter 1.

2. **Weight Gain:** Higher insulin levels can promote fat storage, especially around your abdomen. This weight gain can exacerbate insulin resistance.

3. **Inflammation:** Elevated insulin levels can trigger inflammation in the body, which is associated with a range of health issues.

4. **Type 2 Diabetes:** Prolonged insulin resistance can progress to type 2 diabetes, a condition where your body can't produce enough insulin to control blood sugar effectively.

5. **Heart Health:** High insulin levels can contribute to high blood pressure and unhealthy cholesterol levels, increasing the risk of heart disease.

Conclusion:

In summary, insulin is a critical hormone that acts as a key to unlock your cells' doors and allow glucose in for energy. It's produced by the pancreas and plays a central role in regulating blood sugar levels, maintaining energy balance, and preventing high or low blood sugar extremes.

When insulin doesn't work properly due to insulin resistance, it can lead to a cascade of health issues, including high blood sugar, weight gain, inflammation, and an increased risk of type 2 diabetes and heart disease.

As we move forward in this book, you'll discover how to address insulin resistance through dietary choices, lifestyle adjustments, and more. Understanding insulin's role in your body is the first step toward taking control of your health and managing insulin resistance effectively.

CHAPTER 3

Identifying Insulin Resistance

In the previous chapters, we delved into the intricacies of insulin and how it functions within your body. Now, as we progress in our journey to better understand insulin resistance and how to manage it, Chapter 3 shines a spotlight on the critical topic of identifying insulin resistance. This chapter is all about recognizing the signs, symptoms, and diagnostic methods to detect this condition, paving the way for informed action.

Why Identifying Matters:

Before we dive into the specifics, it's crucial to understand why identifying insulin resistance is so important. Insulin resistance often remains silent in its early stages. This means you might be living with it without even knowing it, all while it quietly wreaks havoc on your health.

The Silent Saboteur:

Imagine you have a saboteur in your body – insulin resistance. It's interfering with your blood sugar control, promoting weight gain, and potentially laying the groundwork for more serious conditions like type 2 diabetes and heart disease. The catch is, it doesn't always come knocking with glaring symptoms.

Common Signs and Symptoms:

Let's explore some common signs and symptoms of insulin resistance that may give you a hint that something's amiss:

1. **Unexplained Fatigue:** If you frequently feel tired, even after a good night's

sleep, it could be related to insulin resistance. Fluctuating blood sugar levels can leave you feeling drained.

2. **Increased Hunger:** Are you always hungry, even shortly after eating a meal? This persistent hunger can be a red flag.

3. **Difficulty Losing Weight:** Despite your best efforts to eat well and exercise, the numbers on the scale refuse to budge, especially around your midsection.

4. **Frequent Urination:** Increased insulin resistance can lead to higher blood sugar levels, causing your kidneys to work harder to remove the excess sugar from your blood. This can result in increased urination.

5. **Dark Skin Patches:** A condition called acanthosis nigricans can manifest as dark, velvety patches of skin, often on the neck, armpits, or groin. It's associated with insulin resistance.

6. **High Blood Pressure:** Elevated insulin levels can contribute to high blood

pressure, which is a risk factor for heart disease.

7. **Abnormal Cholesterol Levels:** Insulin resistance can lead to unhealthy cholesterol profiles, including elevated triglycerides and reduced HDL (the "good" cholesterol).

8. **Polycystic Ovary Syndrome (PCOS):** Women with PCOS often have insulin resistance as a component of their condition. Symptoms may include irregular periods,

acne, and excessive hair growth.

9. **Sleep Troubles:** Insulin resistance can affect sleep patterns, leading to difficulty falling asleep or staying asleep.

10. **Brain Fog:** Some people with insulin resistance report difficulties with concentration and memory, often referred to as "brain fog."

Diagnostic Methods:

If you suspect insulin resistance based on the signs and symptoms mentioned above, it's essential to consult a healthcare professional. They can perform various tests to confirm whether insulin resistance is indeed the issue. Here are some diagnostic methods commonly used:

1. **Fasting Blood Sugar Test:** This test measures your blood sugar level after an overnight fast. If your fasting blood sugar is consistently elevated, it could be an indicator of insulin resistance.

2. **Oral Glucose Tolerance Test (OGTT):** In this test, you'll fast overnight, then

drink a sugary solution. Blood sugar levels are measured at intervals to see how your body processes the glucose load.

3. **Hemoglobin A1c Test:** This test provides a snapshot of your average blood sugar levels over the past few months. It's a valuable tool for identifying long-term blood sugar control.

4. **Insulin Level Measurement:** Sometimes, healthcare providers may directly measure your insulin levels,

as elevated insulin can be a sign of insulin resistance.

5. **Home Glucose Monitoring:** For some individuals, home glucose monitoring may be recommended to track blood sugar levels throughout the day, providing valuable insights into potential insulin resistance.

Consulting a Healthcare Professional:

If you're experiencing any of the signs and symptoms mentioned earlier, or if you have risk factors such as a family history of diabetes, it's crucial to seek professional guidance. Your healthcare provider can assess your specific situation, order appropriate tests, and provide tailored recommendations based on your results.

Early Detection and Prevention:

One of the key takeaways from this chapter is the importance of early detection. Identifying insulin resistance in its early stages allows you to take proactive steps to manage it effectively. Early intervention can help prevent or delay the progression to type 2 diabetes and reduce the risk of associated health complications.

Conclusion:

In summary, Chapter 3 has shed light on the significance of recognizing insulin resistance. While it can often remain silent in its initial stages, being aware of the common signs and symptoms, along with consulting a healthcare professional for appropriate testing, can make all the difference in early detection.

Identifying insulin resistance is the first step towards taking control of your health. It empowers you with knowledge and the opportunity to implement lifestyle changes, dietary adjustments, and, if needed, medical interventions that can help manage insulin resistance effectively. This proactive approach sets the stage for the chapters to come, where we'll explore strategies to address and even reverse insulin resistance, ultimately improving your overall well-being.

CHAPTER 4

Building an Insulin-Friendly Diet

In our exploration of the journey to understand and manage insulin resistance, we've already covered the fundamentals of insulin, its role in the body, and how to identify the signs of insulin resistance. Now, we step into Chapter 4, where we'll delve into the heart of the matter: building an insulin-friendly diet. This chapter is your guide to making food choices that can help manage insulin resistance effectively.

The Power of Diet:

Diet plays a central role in managing insulin resistance. The foods you eat can directly impact your blood sugar levels and insulin response. Crafting an insulin-friendly diet involves making choices that promote stable blood sugar levels and reduce the need for excessive insulin production.

Balancing Macronutrients:

One of the fundamental principles of an insulin-friendly diet is finding the right balance of macronutrients − carbohydrates, protein, and fat. Let's break down how each of these components influences insulin and blood sugar:

1. Carbohydrates: Carbohydrates are a primary source of glucose, which has the most significant impact on blood sugar levels. However, not all carbs are created equal.

- **Simple Carbs:** These are found in sugary foods and processed grains. They cause rapid spikes in blood sugar and should be limited.

- **Complex Carbs:** These are found in whole grains, vegetables, and legumes. They provide a slower, more sustained release of glucose, promoting stable blood sugar levels.

2. **Protein:** Protein-rich foods like lean meats, fish, and plant-based sources (e.g., beans and tofu) have a relatively modest impact on blood sugar. They also help you feel full, reducing the likelihood of overeating.

3. **Fat:** Healthy fats from sources like avocados, nuts, seeds, and olive oil can further slow the

absorption of glucose from your meals. This can help prevent rapid spikes in blood sugar.

Fiber: Your Insulin-Friendly Ally:

Fiber is an unsung hero in the quest for an insulin-friendly diet. It's found in plant-based foods like fruits, vegetables, whole grains, legumes, and nuts. Here's why fiber is crucial:

1. **Slows Digestion:** Fiber-rich foods take longer to digest, leading to a gradual release of glucose into the bloodstream. This helps

prevent sudden blood sugar spikes.

2. **Promotes Fullness:** Foods high in fiber help you feel full and satisfied, reducing the urge to overeat or snack on less healthy options.

3. **Improved Gut Health:** Fiber is essential for a healthy gut microbiome, which has been linked to better blood sugar control.

Managing Carbohydrates:

Since carbohydrates have the most significant impact on blood sugar, managing them is a key component of an insulin-friendly diet. Here are some strategies:

1. **Choose Whole Grains:** Opt for whole grains like brown rice, quinoa, and whole wheat bread instead of refined grains like white rice and white bread.

2. **Mind Your Portions:** Be mindful of portion sizes, especially when it comes to carbohydrate-rich foods. This can help prevent excessive glucose spikes.

3. **Favor Low-Glycemic Foods:** The glycemic index (GI) ranks foods based on

their impact on blood sugar. Lower-GI foods, like sweet potatoes and legumes, are less likely to cause rapid blood sugar spikes.

4. **Balanced Meals:** Create balanced meals that include carbohydrates, protein, and healthy fats. This combination helps stabilize blood sugar levels.

The Importance of Meal Timing:

When you eat can be just as important as what you eat. Spacing your meals throughout the day and avoiding long periods without food can help maintain stable blood sugar levels. Consider these meal timing tips:

1. **Regular Meals:** Aim for three balanced meals a day with healthy snacks if needed. Skipping meals can lead to blood sugar fluctuations.

2. **Don't Skip Breakfast:** Breakfast kickstarts your metabolism and provides essential energy after an overnight fast.

3. **Avoid Late-Night Eating:** Eating large meals late at night can disrupt your

body's natural blood sugar rhythm.

4. **Consider Intermittent Fasting:** Some individuals with insulin resistance benefit from intermittent fasting, which involves cycling between periods of eating and fasting.

Glycemic Load vs. Glycemic Index:

Understanding the glycemic load (GL) of foods can be more informative than just considering their glycemic index. The glycemic load takes into account both the quality and quantity of carbohydrates in a food.

- **High GL:** Foods with a high GL have a significant impact on blood sugar. These should be consumed in moderation.

- **Low GL:** Foods with a low GL have a minimal effect on blood sugar and are generally better choices.

The Role of Sugar and Sweeteners:

Reducing added sugars in your diet is paramount for managing insulin resistance. These sugars can quickly send your blood sugar levels soaring. Consider these steps:

1. **Limit Added Sugars:** Read food labels to identify added sugars in products and reduce your consumption of sugary beverages, candies, and sweets.

2. **Natural Sweeteners:** If you need sweetness, consider using natural sweeteners like stevia or erythritol, which have a lower impact on blood sugar.

The Mediterranean Diet Approach:

The Mediterranean diet is often recommended for individuals with insulin resistance. It emphasizes:

- Abundant vegetables and fruits.
- Whole grains.
- Healthy fats like olive oil and nuts.
- Lean protein sources like fish and legumes.
- Moderate alcohol consumption (typically red wine).
- Limited red meat and processed foods.

Hydration Matters:

Don't forget about hydration. Water is essential for overall health, including blood sugar regulation. Aim to drink plenty of water throughout the day.

Consulting a Registered Dietitian:

While these dietary guidelines provide a solid foundation for managing insulin resistance, it's crucial to recognize that individual needs vary. Consulting a registered dietitian can provide personalized guidance tailored to your specific situation. They can help you create a meal plan that works for you, taking into account your preferences, lifestyle, and any other health conditions you may have.

In Conclusion:

Chapter 4 has unveiled the principles of an insulin-friendly diet, focusing on the importance of macronutrient balance, fiber, meal timing, and glycemic load. Your dietary choices have a direct impact on blood sugar levels and insulin response, making informed decisions about what you eat a powerful tool in managing insulin resistance.

As we move forward in this journey, we'll explore other lifestyle strategies, exercise, and ways to enhance your overall well-being while effectively managing insulin resistance. Remember, small changes in your diet can lead to significant improvements in your health, making each meal an opportunity for positive change.

CHAPTER 5

Incorporating Whole Foods

Chapter 5 of our exploration into managing insulin resistance takes us into the world of whole foods. Understanding and incorporating whole foods into your diet is a fundamental aspect of an insulin-friendly eating plan. In this chapter, we'll delve into the significance of whole foods, why they matter in managing insulin resistance, and how to make them a delicious and satisfying part of your daily meals.

What Are Whole Foods?

Whole foods are foods that are as close to their natural state as possible. They are minimally processed or refined, and they contain no added sugars, preservatives, or artificial additives. Whole foods include fruits, vegetables, whole grains, legumes, nuts, seeds, lean proteins, and unprocessed dairy products.

The Whole Food Advantage:

Whole foods provide several advantages when it comes to managing insulin resistance:

1. **Nutrient Density:** Whole foods are packed with essential vitamins, minerals, fiber, and antioxidants. They offer a wide range of nutrients that support overall health and help regulate blood sugar.

2. **Fiber Content:** As mentioned in the previous chapter, fiber plays a pivotal role in stabilizing blood sugar levels. Whole foods are rich in dietary fiber,

promoting a gradual release of glucose into the bloodstream.

3. **Slow Digestion:** Whole foods are digested more slowly than processed foods, leading to a steady and sustained supply of energy. This prevents rapid spikes and crashes in blood sugar levels.

4. **Satiety:** Whole foods are often more filling and satisfying, reducing the temptation to overeat or snack on unhealthy options.

Incorporating Whole Foods:

Now, let's explore how to incorporate more whole foods into your diet to effectively manage insulin resistance:

1. Start with Vegetables:

Vegetables are the cornerstone of a whole-foods-based diet. They are low in calories, high in fiber, and loaded with essential nutrients. Aim to fill half your plate with non-starchy vegetables like leafy greens, broccoli, cauliflower, bell peppers, and zucchini.

2. Choose Whole Grains:

When selecting grains, opt for whole grains like brown rice, quinoa, whole wheat pasta, and oats. These grains are less processed and retain their bran and germ, which contain valuable fiber and nutrients.

3. Embrace Legumes:

Legumes, such as beans, lentils, and chickpeas, are excellent sources of plant-based protein and fiber. They can be used in soups, stews, salads, and even blended into dips like hummus.

4. Include Lean Proteins:

Incorporate lean protein sources like skinless poultry, fish, tofu, and tempeh. Protein helps stabilize blood sugar levels and keeps you feeling full.

5. Snack on Nuts and Seeds:

Nuts and seeds, such as almonds, walnuts, chia seeds, and flaxseeds, are nutritious snacks that provide healthy fats, fiber, and protein. A small handful of nuts makes for a satisfying and insulin-friendly snack.

6. Enjoy Fresh Fruits:

While fruits do contain natural sugars, they are also rich in fiber, vitamins, and antioxidants. Choose a variety of colorful fruits and consume them in moderation as part of a balanced diet.

7. Limit Processed Foods:

Processed foods are often laden with refined sugars, unhealthy fats, and additives that can disrupt blood sugar control. Minimize your intake of items like sugary cereals, packaged snacks, and sugary beverages.

8. Cook at Home:

Preparing meals at home gives you control over the ingredients you use. It allows you to choose whole foods and avoid the hidden sugars and unhealthy fats often found in restaurant or takeout meals.

9. Read Food Labels:

When buying packaged foods, read labels carefully. Look for products with simple, recognizable ingredients and minimal added sugars.

10. Hydrate with Water:

Water is the best choice for staying hydrated. Avoid sugary drinks like sodas and many fruit juices, as they can lead to blood sugar spikes.

Whole Food-Based Meal Ideas:

Creating whole food-based meals can be both nutritious and delicious. Here are some meal ideas to inspire your insulin-friendly diet:

1. Breakfast:

- Overnight oats made with rolled oats, almond milk, chia seeds, and berries.
- Scrambled eggs with spinach, mushrooms, and whole-grain toast.
- Greek yogurt topped with sliced almonds, fresh fruit,

and a drizzle of honey (in moderation).

2. Lunch:

- Quinoa salad with mixed vegetables, chickpeas, and a lemon-tahini dressing.
- Grilled chicken breast with a side of steamed broccoli and brown rice.
- Lentil soup with a side of mixed greens.

3. Dinner:

- Baked salmon with roasted sweet potatoes and asparagus.

- Stir-fried tofu with mixed vegetables and quinoa.
- Stuffed bell peppers with lean ground turkey, brown rice, and diced tomatoes.

4. Snacks:

- Carrot and cucumber sticks with hummus.
- A small handful of mixed nuts.
- Sliced apple with almond butter.

Remember Portion Control:

While whole foods are nutritious, portion control is still important, especially if you're trying to manage your weight. Even healthy foods can contribute to weight gain if consumed in excessive amounts.

Consulting a Registered Dietitian:

As with any dietary changes, it's beneficial to consult a registered dietitian. They can create a personalized meal plan tailored to your needs and help you navigate the world of whole foods, ensuring that your diet supports your goals for managing insulin resistance.

In Conclusion:

Chapter 5 has illuminated the significance of incorporating whole foods into your diet to effectively manage insulin resistance. Whole foods are nutrient-dense, fiber-rich, and promote stable blood sugar levels. They also offer a wide range of delicious and satisfying meal options that can help you maintain a healthy and balanced eating pattern.

Remember that building an insulin-friendly diet is a gradual process. Small changes in your food choices can yield significant benefits for your health. As we move forward in this journey, we'll explore additional lifestyle strategies, including exercise and stress management, to enhance your overall well-being while effectively managing insulin resistance.

CHAPTER 6

Managing Carbohydrates

In Chapter 6 of our exploration into managing insulin resistance, we're diving deep into the world of carbohydrates. Understanding how to manage carbohydrates effectively is a pivotal aspect of an insulin-friendly diet. This chapter will elucidate the role of carbohydrates in blood sugar control, explain the concept of glycemic index and load, and provide practical strategies for incorporating carbohydrates in a way that supports insulin sensitivity.

Carbohydrates: The Double-Edged Sword:

Carbohydrates are a double-edged sword when it comes to insulin resistance. On one hand, they are a primary source of glucose, which can lead to spikes in blood sugar levels. On the other hand, they are an essential nutrient that provides energy and a range of vital nutrients, including fiber, vitamins, and minerals.

The Glycemic Index (GI):

To understand the impact of carbohydrates on blood sugar, we turn to the concept of the glycemic index (GI). The GI is a scale that ranks carbohydrate-containing foods based on how quickly they raise blood sugar levels compared to pure glucose, which has a GI of 100. Foods with a higher GI cause a more rapid increase in blood sugar.

High-GI vs. Low-GI Foods:

- **High-GI Foods:** These include foods like white bread, sugary cereals, and most processed snack foods. They cause a quick spike in blood sugar levels, followed by a crash, which can leave you feeling hungry and irritable shortly after eating.

- **Low-GI Foods:** These are foods that have a slower and more gradual impact on blood sugar. Examples include whole grains, legumes, non-starchy vegetables, and many fruits. They provide a steady supply of energy and help maintain stable blood sugar levels.

The Glycemic Load (GL):

While the GI is a useful tool, it doesn't tell the whole story. It doesn't account for portion sizes. Enter the glycemic load (GL). The GL takes both the quality and quantity of carbohydrates into account. It provides a more accurate picture of how a particular food will affect blood sugar.

- **High-GL Foods:** These are foods that not only have a high GI but are also consumed in large quantities. A good example is watermelon. While it has a high GI, you'd have to eat a substantial amount to significantly impact blood sugar.

- **Low-GL Foods:** These are foods that have a lower GI and are typically consumed in reasonable portions. Most non-starchy vegetables, for instance, have a low GL.

Strategies for Managing Carbohydrates:

Now that we've covered the basics of GI and GL, let's explore practical strategies for managing carbohydrates effectively when dealing with insulin resistance:

1. Choose Whole Grains:

Opt for whole grains like brown rice, quinoa, whole wheat pasta, and oats. These grains are less processed and contain more fiber, vitamins, and minerals compared to their refined counterparts.

2. Mind Your Portions:

Be mindful of portion sizes, especially when it comes to carbohydrate-rich foods like grains, starchy vegetables, and fruits. Keeping portions in check can help prevent excessive glucose spikes.

3. Balance Your Plate:

Create balanced meals that include carbohydrates, protein, and healthy fats. This combination helps slow down the digestion of carbohydrates, preventing rapid blood sugar fluctuations.

4. Include Fiber-Rich Foods:

Foods high in dietary fiber, such as non-starchy vegetables, legumes, and whole fruits, can help stabilize blood sugar levels. Aim to include them in each meal.

5. Don't Skip Meals:

Skipping meals can lead to erratic blood sugar levels. Ensure you have regular, balanced meals and consider healthy snacks if needed to avoid long periods without food.

6. Limit Sugary and Processed Foods:

Processed foods and those high in added sugars can cause rapid blood sugar spikes. Minimize your intake of sugary cereals, candies, and sweets.

7. Experiment with Low-GI and Low-GL Foods:

Explore low-GI and low-GL foods in your diet. These options can help maintain steady blood sugar levels. Examples include lentils, chickpeas, quinoa, and most non-starchy vegetables.

8. Pay Attention to Meal Timing:

The timing of your carbohydrate intake matters. Consuming carbohydrates earlier in the day when your body is more insulin-sensitive can help regulate blood sugar more effectively.

9. Monitor Your Blood Sugar:

If you have insulin resistance or diabetes, your healthcare provider may recommend monitoring your blood sugar levels regularly. This can provide valuable insights into how specific foods and meals affect your body.

10. Customize Your Diet:

Remember that everyone's tolerance for carbohydrates varies. What works for one person may not work for another. Personalize your carbohydrate intake based on your body's response and consult a registered dietitian for tailored guidance.

Glycemic Index and Food Combining:

Food combining is another approach that some individuals with insulin resistance find beneficial. It involves pairing carbohydrates with protein or healthy fats to slow down their digestion and reduce their impact on blood sugar.

For example, instead of eating a plain bagel (high-GI), you might top it with almond butter (protein and healthy fat) to mitigate its glycemic effect.

The Importance of Fiber:

Fiber is a dietary superhero when it comes to managing insulin resistance. It not only slows down the digestion of carbohydrates but also promotes fullness and helps control appetite. Fiber-rich foods like vegetables, legumes, whole grains, and nuts should be a staple in your diet.

Consulting a Registered Dietitian:

As always, consulting a registered dietitian is highly recommended, especially when managing insulin resistance. They can help you create a personalized meal plan that considers your specific needs, preferences, and tolerance for carbohydrates.

In Conclusion:

Chapter 6 has delved into the intricate world of managing carbohydrates to effectively control blood sugar levels in the context of insulin resistance. By understanding the glycemic index, glycemic load, and applying practical strategies like choosing whole grains, balancing meals, and monitoring portion sizes, you can navigate the complexities of carbohydrates successfully.

Remember that managing insulin resistance through dietary choices is a journey. Experimentation, patience, and professional guidance can help you find the right approach that suits your body and supports your overall health and well-being. In the chapters ahead, we'll continue to explore additional lifestyle strategies and insights to empower you on your path to managing insulin resistance effectively.

CHAPTER 7

The Role of Exercise

Chapter 7 of our journey through managing insulin resistance introduces the powerful influence of exercise on this condition. Regular physical activity is a cornerstone of a healthy lifestyle and plays a crucial role in improving insulin sensitivity, blood sugar control, and overall well-being. In this chapter, we will explore the mechanisms by which exercise benefits those with insulin resistance and provide practical guidance on incorporating physical activity into your daily routine.

The Insulin-Exercise Connection:

Exercise and insulin resistance are intertwined in a fascinating way. When you engage in physical activity, several beneficial changes occur in your body:

1. Improved Insulin Sensitivity: Regular exercise enhances the ability of your cells to respond to insulin. This means your body can use insulin more effectively to transport glucose into your cells for energy.

2. Blood Sugar Regulation:

Exercise helps regulate blood sugar levels by increasing the uptake of glucose by muscle cells. This reduces the reliance on insulin to keep blood sugar in check.

3. Weight Management:

Physical activity contributes to weight loss or weight maintenance, which is vital for improving insulin sensitivity. Excess body fat, especially around the abdomen, is closely linked to insulin resistance.

4. Muscle Glucose Uptake: When you exercise, your muscles use glucose for energy. This process doesn't require insulin, making it an efficient way to lower blood sugar levels.

5. Enhanced Cardiovascular Health: Exercise has numerous cardiovascular benefits, including lowering blood pressure and improving cholesterol profiles. People with insulin resistance are often at higher risk for heart disease, so these improvements are especially important.

Types of Exercise:

Effective exercise for managing insulin resistance encompasses various types, each offering unique benefits:

1. **Aerobic Exercise:** Also known as cardio, this type of exercise gets your heart rate up and includes activities like walking, jogging, cycling, swimming, and dancing. Aerobic exercise enhances insulin sensitivity, burns calories, and supports cardiovascular health.

2. **Strength Training:** Resistance or strength training involves lifting weights or using resistance bands to build and

strengthen muscles. This type of exercise helps increase muscle mass, which can lead to improved blood sugar control.

3. High-Intensity Interval Training (HIIT): HIIT involves short bursts of intense exercise followed by brief rest periods. It's efficient and effective for improving both cardiovascular fitness and insulin sensitivity.

4. Flexibility and Balance Exercises: Activities like yoga and Pilates improve flexibility, balance, and overall body awareness. They can be valuable additions to your exercise routine, helping to prevent injuries.

5. Everyday Physical Activity:

Don't forget about the value of everyday movement. Activities like gardening, housework, and taking the stairs can all contribute to your daily exercise.

Frequency and Duration:

For those with insulin resistance, the American Diabetes Association recommends:

- At least 150 minutes of moderate-intensity aerobic exercise per week, spread over at least three days.

- Resistance training at least two days per week.

Remember, consistency is key. Regular exercise yields the most significant benefits in terms of improving insulin sensitivity.

Finding the Right Exercise Routine:

The ideal exercise routine is one that you enjoy and can maintain over the long term. Here are some tips for finding the right fit:

1. **Start Slowly:** If you're new to exercise or haven't been active for a while, start with manageable goals. Gradually increase the

intensity and duration as your fitness improves.

2. Mix It Up: Variety can make exercise more enjoyable and prevent boredom. Try different types of activities to keep things interesting.

3. Listen to Your Body: Pay attention to how your body responds to exercise. If you experience pain or discomfort, adjust your routine accordingly and consider consulting a fitness professional.

4. Set Realistic Goals: Set achievable goals that are specific, measurable, and time-bound. This can help keep you motivated and on track.

5. Seek Support: Consider working with a fitness trainer or joining a group exercise class. Having support and guidance can make exercise more enjoyable and effective.

6. Prioritize Safety: Safety should always come first. If you have any underlying health conditions or concerns, consult your healthcare provider before starting a new exercise program.

Combining Exercise with Diet:

Exercise and diet work synergistically in managing insulin resistance. When you combine an insulin-friendly diet with regular physical activity, you maximize your chances of success. Here's how they complement each other:

- Diet influences your baseline blood sugar and insulin levels.
- Exercise helps your cells become more sensitive to insulin and burn glucose efficiently.

- Together, they support weight management, which is critical for improving insulin sensitivity.

Blood Sugar Monitoring:

If you have insulin resistance, particularly if you're on medication or insulin therapy, monitoring your blood sugar before and after exercise can be valuable. It helps you understand how different types and durations of exercise affect your blood sugar levels.

Pre-Exercise: Check your blood sugar levels before exercise. If they're low, have a small snack to prevent hypoglycemia (low blood sugar).

Post-Exercise: Monitor your blood sugar after exercise to see how your body responds. It's common for blood sugar to drop after physical activity. If it drops excessively, adjust your pre-exercise snack or insulin doses as advised by your healthcare provider.

Stress Management and Sleep:

In the context of managing insulin resistance, stress management and adequate sleep are often overlooked but crucial factors. Chronic stress and poor sleep can contribute to insulin resistance and blood sugar dysregulation.

- **Stress Management:** Techniques like mindfulness meditation, deep breathing exercises, and progressive muscle relaxation can help reduce stress levels.
- **Sleep:** Aim for 7-9 hours of quality sleep per night. Poor sleep can disrupt hormones that regulate appetite and blood sugar.

Consulting a Healthcare Professional:

Before embarking on a new exercise program, especially if you have underlying health conditions, it's essential to consult your healthcare provider. They can assess your specific situation, provide guidance on exercise safety, and tailor recommendations to your needs.

In Conclusion:

Chapter 7 has illuminated the pivotal role of exercise in managing insulin resistance. Regular physical activity improves insulin sensitivity, regulates blood sugar, supports weight management, and enhances overall health. The types and duration of exercise should align with your fitness level and preferences, and consistency is key to reaping the benefits.

By combining an insulin-friendly diet with a well-rounded exercise routine, along with managing stress and ensuring adequate sleep, you can effectively manage insulin resistance and enhance your overall well-being. This holistic approach empowers you to take control of your health and enjoy a vibrant, active life.

CHAPTER 8

Lifestyle for Long-Term Success

As we reach the final chapter of our journey on managing insulin resistance, we arrive at a critical point – maintaining long-term success. While the previous chapters have provided insights into the role of insulin, dietary choices, exercise, and various strategies for managing this condition, this chapter focuses on how to integrate these principles into a sustainable and fulfilling lifestyle.

The Challenge of Long-Term Success:

Maintaining a healthy lifestyle over the long term can be challenging. Life is dynamic, and various factors, including work, family, and unexpected events, can disrupt even the most well-structured plans. However, the key to successfully managing insulin resistance lies in consistency, adaptability, and balance.

Consistency Is Key:

Consistency is the bedrock of managing insulin resistance. Sustainable changes in diet and exercise, supported by stress management and good sleep habits, form the basis of a long-term strategy.

1. Diet Consistency: Commit to making insulin-friendly dietary choices a consistent part of your life. This doesn't mean perfection but rather a pattern of making better choices most of the time. Enjoy occasional treats, but remember that moderation is crucial.

2. Exercise Routine: Find an exercise routine that you genuinely enjoy and can maintain. Consistency here is essential for improving insulin sensitivity and overall fitness. Adjust your routine as needed to keep it engaging.

3. Stress Management: Incorporate stress management techniques into your daily routine. This could be as simple as a few minutes of deep breathing exercises or mindfulness meditation. Consistency in managing stress contributes to better overall health.

4. Sleep Hygiene: Prioritize good sleep hygiene habits. Maintain a regular sleep schedule, create a comfortable sleep environment, and unwind before bedtime. Consistent sleep patterns support hormonal balance and overall well-being.

Adaptability:

Flexibility is vital for long-term success. Life's demands and circumstances can change, so your approach to managing insulin resistance may need to evolve as well.

1. Adapt to Life Changes: If your work or family responsibilities change, be prepared to adjust your diet and exercise routines accordingly. A new job or a new addition to the family may necessitate modifications.

2. Listen to Your Body: Pay attention to how your body responds to dietary choices and exercise. Over time, your body's needs may change. Be open to adjusting your strategies based on what works best for you.

3. Seek Support: Don't hesitate to reach out for support from healthcare professionals, registered dietitians, or fitness trainers if needed. They can help you adapt your approach to changing circumstances.

Balance:

Long-term success also requires balance. It's essential to balance the various aspects of your life while managing insulin resistance effectively.

1. Work-Life Balance: Strive for a healthy work-life balance. Managing stress and ensuring adequate sleep often start with setting boundaries in your professional life.

2. Enjoy Life: Don't forget to enjoy life. It's perfectly okay to indulge in occasional treats or special occasions. Balance is about finding a middle ground between managing your health and enjoying the pleasures of life.

3. Social Connections: Maintain social connections and relationships. Social support is essential for emotional well-being and can help you stay motivated in your journey.

4. Self-Compassion: Be kind to yourself. Managing insulin resistance can be challenging, and there will be ups and downs. Instead of berating yourself for slip-ups, practice self-compassion and get back on track.

5. Monitor and Reflect: Periodically monitor your progress and reflect on your journey. Celebrate your successes, learn from your setbacks, and adjust your strategies as needed to stay on course.

Setting Realistic Goals:

Realistic and achievable goals are crucial for long-term success. Set yourself up for sustainable progress by creating SMART goals:

- **Specific:** Clearly define what you want to achieve.
- **Measurable:** Use quantifiable criteria to track your progress.
- **Achievable:** Make sure your goals are realistic and within reach.
- **Relevant:** Ensure your goals are relevant to your long-term health.

- **Time-Bound:** Set a timeline for when you aim to achieve your goals.

Here's an example of a SMART goal: "I will walk for 30 minutes, five days a week, for the next three months to improve my fitness and blood sugar control."

Celebrate Your Achievements:

Recognize and celebrate your achievements, no matter how small. Each milestone, whether it's losing a few pounds, consistently sticking to your exercise routine, or successfully managing stress, deserves acknowledgment. Celebrating your progress can boost motivation and reinforce positive habits.

Support Systems:

Having a support system in place can significantly contribute to long-term success. This support can come from various sources:

- **Healthcare Professionals:** Regular check-ins with your healthcare provider or registered dietitian can help you stay on track and make necessary adjustments to your plan.

- **Family and Friends:** Share your goals and progress with your loved ones. They can provide encouragement and accountability.

- **Support Groups:** Consider joining a support group or online community for individuals managing insulin resistance or similar health conditions. Sharing experiences and advice can be empowering.

The Power of Mindset:

Your mindset plays a pivotal role in long-term success. Cultivate a growth mindset, which embraces challenges as opportunities for growth and learning. A growth mindset can help you navigate setbacks and maintain a positive outlook on your journey.

Seek Professional Guidance:

If you ever feel overwhelmed or uncertain about managing insulin resistance, don't hesitate to seek professional guidance. Healthcare providers, registered dietitians, and fitness trainers have the knowledge and expertise to provide tailored recommendations that align with your unique needs and circumstances.

In Conclusion:

Chapter 8, the final chapter of our exploration into managing insulin resistance, underscores the importance of adopting a lifestyle that fosters long-term success. Consistency, adaptability, and balance are the cornerstones of this lifestyle, enabling you to navigate life's challenges while effectively managing insulin resistance.

Remember that managing insulin resistance is a journey, not a destination. By incorporating the principles from this journey – understanding insulin, making wise dietary choices, engaging in regular exercise, managing stress, prioritizing sleep, and fostering a growth mindset – you empower yourself to lead a healthier, more fulfilling life. Stay committed to your well-being, and embrace each day as an opportunity to make choices that support your health and happiness.

In the culmination of our exploration into managing insulin resistance, we've embarked on a transformative journey toward better health and well-being. This book has guided us through eight comprehensive chapters, each offering valuable insights and practical strategies for understanding, controlling, and thriving despite insulin resistance.

We began by demystifying insulin, unveiling its pivotal role in our bodies and how it can sometimes become a double-edged sword. We then delved into the intricate realm of dietary choices, uncovering the power of whole foods, balanced macronutrients, and the importance of meal timing.

Our journey continued with an exploration of carbohydrates, unravelling the mysteries of the glycemic index and load, and learning how to make informed choices to keep blood sugar levels stable. We then turned our attention to the significant role of exercise in improving insulin sensitivity, cardiovascular health, and overall vitality.

Throughout this voyage, we discovered that managing insulin resistance is not a solitary endeavor; it's a holistic lifestyle. Stress management and quality sleep were revealed as critical factors often overlooked in the quest for better health.

CONCLUSION

Finally, we wrapped up our journey in Chapter 8, where we explored the principles of consistency, adaptability, and balance that are vital for long-term success. We emphasized that while life may present challenges, adopting a growth mindset and seeking support from professionals and loved ones can keep us on the path to better health.

As we conclude this book, remember that managing insulin resistance is a lifelong journey. It's about more than just controlling blood sugar levels; it's about nurturing a vibrant, fulfilling life. Every step you take, every choice you make, contributes to your overall well-being.

In this concluding moment, let's reaffirm the central message of our journey: Empowerment. You have the knowledge, tools, and capacity to manage insulin resistance effectively. By making informed choices, embracing a balanced lifestyle, and seeking support when needed, you can enhance your quality of life and live well despite the challenges posed by this condition.

May this book serve as a valuable companion on your path to health and vitality. As you continue your journey, remember that your health is an investment, not an expense, and the choices you make today will shape the health you enjoy tomorrow. Here's to a future filled with well-being, resilience, and the empowerment to thrive, no matter what challenges may come your way.

9 798867 775711